KT-369-728

THE <u>NEW</u> SELF HELP SERIES

HIGH BLOOD PRESSURE

by
LEON CHAITOW
N.D., D.O.

THORSONS PUBLISHING GROUP

First published April 1986

British Library Cataloguing in Publication Data

Chaitow, Leon
High blood-pressure.
1. Hypertension—Treatment
I. Title
616.1'3206   RC685.H8

ISBN 0-7225-1221-X

Published by Thorsons Publishers Limited,
Wellingborough, Northamptonshire, NN8 2RQ,
England

Printed in Great Britain by
Richard Clay Limited, Bungay, Suffolk.

7 9 10 8 6

THE <u>NEW</u> SELF HELP SERIES

HIGH BLOOD PRESSURE

A naturopathic practitioner provides advice on this
all-too-common problem and provides a programme
of self-help, natural remedies.

Contents

Note to reader

Before following the self-help advice given in this book readers are earnestly urged to give careful consideration to the nature of their particular health problem, and to consult a competent physician if in any doubt. This book should not be regarded as a substitute for professional medical treatment, and whilst every care is taken to ensure the accuracy of the content, the author and the publishers cannot accept legal responsibility for any problem arising out of the experimentation with the methods described.

This book is for Sasha

INTRODUCTION

What is Blood-Pressure?

The aim of this book is for you to come to a general understanding of your body, and your blood-pressure in particular, as it relates to your health and your life. In so doing you will achieve insights into the marvellous manner in which the body functions and how it is possible for problems to arise in the cardio-vascular system which are directly related to factors over which you have a good degree of control. Hypertension, or as it commonly called high blood-pressure, is one indication of problems arising. It is not a disease as such but it is a condition which can be life endangering, and is in fact the leading contributory cause of death in the industrialized countries of the West.

We will look at the dynamics of the cardio-vascular system, and just how blood-pressure relates to health; we will investigate the major factors in our lifestyles and diets that can influence it, and above all we will delve into the ways in which problems can be avoided and overcome in this regard. There is growing realization, in the medical world, that it is necessary for there to be a change in attitude towards disease, away from the idea that there is a 'cure' for everything, via drugs or treatment, and towards the concept of individuals taking personal responsibility for the maintenance and regaining of health. Nowhere is this more true than in the area of hypertension, where simple alterations in diet, exercise and behaviour, can often dramatically change a situation in which there is real danger, to one in which healthy function is restored.

If you want to understand what blood-pressure is all about, what high blood-pressure results from, and its implications; and what you, yourself, can do to avoid or reverse such a problem, then this book is designed for you.

It is not suggested that medical treatment of hypertension is always unnecessary, but it is suggested that drug treatment is frequently used when self-help methods would provide a better and safer long-term solution.

The Circulatory System

Picture the following sequence of events, which takes place within the closed circuit of the circulatory system of the body. The muscular pump, the heart, receives via the venous system blood which requires cleansing of its load of carbon dioxide (picked up as the blood passed through the body) and it pumps this to the lungs where the blood will detoxify and collect fresh oxygen for the use of the body. This oxygenated blood returns to the heart, from the lungs, and is pumped into the arteries. These have a degree of elasticity, and stretch to accommodate the blood as it is pumped into them.

The amount of pressure in the artery at the moment

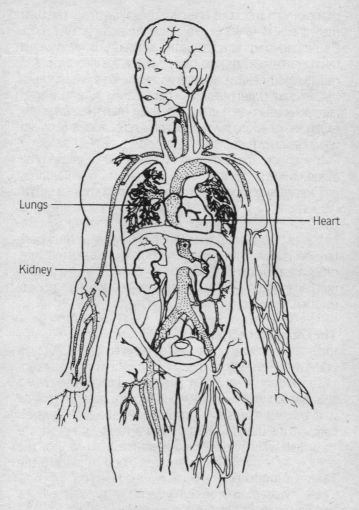

Lungs

Heart

Kidney

Figure 1: **The circulatory system**

of maximum effort of the heart (as it beats) is the first measurement taken when blood-pressure is recorded. This is called systolic pressure. Pressure is maintained by the artery after the beat, whilst the heart muscle relaxes momentarily before its next effort.

The amount of pressure registered during this brief rest phase, between beats, is the other measurement taken when recording blood-pressure, and it is called the diastolic pressure. This is the lowest pressure found in the arterial system after the heart has pumped the blood into it.

The pressure rises again as the heart pumps again. As we will see, anything that increases the overall pressure on the arterial system, will result in the diastolic pressure being increased. This can involve a number of possible factors, including the loss of elasticity in the blood-vessel walls, through hardening, or increased muscular pressure resulting from stressed or tensed muscles pressing on them. Such increased pressure in the blood-vessels results in the heart having to pump harder in order to force the blood through them, and the end result of this could reflect in the systolic pressure reading as well.

To summarize what has been said above: the forceful moment of blood being pumped into the arterial system is the systolic pressure, and the rest phase, between beats, when the actual inter-arterial pressure is recorded, is the diastolic pressure.

Taking Blood-Pressure

These pressures are measured by an instrument called a sphygmomanometer. Using an air-filled cuff it occludes, or cuts off, the circulation momentarily whilst the sound

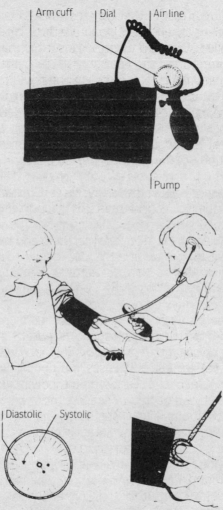

Figure 2: **Testing blood-pressure**

of the pulses is listened for by means of either a stethoscope or an electronic device. As the heart pumps, the air in the cuff is slowly released until the pressure of the heart matches the pressure of the cuff of the sphygmomanometer, the sound of the pulse heard at that moment signals the systolic level, on a column of mercury. As the heart effort eases, during the rest between beats, the level of mercury drops in its column, and the next 'sound' listened for is that of the cessation of the sound of the pulsation of blood through the artery as the cuff releases its pressure on it. This is the actual pressure level in the artery, also expressed by the height of the column of mercury, supported by the pressure.

The readings thus taken are recorded, and these are written, or stated, as the systolic figure 'over' the diastolic figure. In a normal, average, individual, this would be around 120 over 80 (120/80) millimetres of mercury (mm/Hg).

From these two figures much can be deduced about the health of the individual. It should be noted that these figures represent the pressure of blood when the measurement is taken at the usual position of the upper arm, at the level of the heart, with the individual seated, and the arm supported. The pressure will vary in different positions (lying, standing) and in different locations (upper or lower leg, etc.).

It is possible for great variations to exist in pressures, under varying conditions, and in different positions, and for important diagnostic information to be gathered in this way. However, it is the commonly taken arm pressure that we are referring to, in this instance, as being 'normal' at 120/80/mm/Hg.

It is also worth noting that apprehension or slight tension on the part of the person having their pressure taken can alter the accuracy of the reading quite markedly. Thus it has been suggested that the pressure should be taken at least twice, and preferably three times over a fifteen minute period, and the last one of all taken as being the most accurate, if the 'anxiety' factor is to be avoided. It was noted, in an Italian trial, that hospital patients about to have their pressure recorded showed an increase in diastolic pressure which was maintained for ten minutes or more. Thus the practice was introduced of taking the pressure several times, and leaving the sphygmomanometer cuff in position all the while, to overcome the anxiety felt about the procedure.

How Blood Circulation Works

The pumping of the heart (over 100,000 contractions daily) starts the blood on its journey which takes it through a maze of over 60,000 miles of networked vessels. All those carrying fresh, oxygen-rich blood are directed away from the heart, and all those returning 'used' blood for reprocessing (the veins and venules) run towards the heart. The veins, which frequently have to carry blood against the force of gravity, have one-way valves to prevent blood from becoming stagnant, or actually passing the wrong way. It is certainly not possible for the heart action to have the power to pump all the blood, all the way around this vast network of tubes, and it is important that we realize that muscular activity, and the action of breathing, have a vital role to play in the whole process of circulation, for these factors are keys to assisting in blood-pressure problems.

Arteries

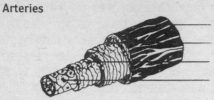

Outer coating
Muscle
Elastic tissue
Inner lining

Veins

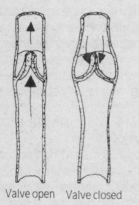

Valve open   Valve closed

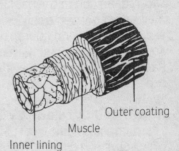

Outer coating
Muscle
Inner lining

Capillaries
Oxygen and
nutrients pass
through
capillary wall

Figure 3: **The structure of the blood vessels**

One of the most important parts of the circulatory network are the tiny, often microscopically fine, arterioles. These are the network of vessels which carry fresh blood to every part of the body, having branched off from the arteries proper. These have a coating of muscle which is directly under the control of the nervous system, and which helps to regulate the activity of the blood distribution system. As these arterioles deliver their oxygenated blood, tiny venules collect used blood for return to the heart. These, like tributaries to a river, join together to form large veins which depend on two vast systems of pumps for the movement of the blood they contain. The first is the muscle pump system. Every time a muscle is used, it contracts. As it does so veins that lie within it are squeezed. Since they have one-way valves this moves the contents forward (towards the heart).

A vast reservoir of blood moving towards the heart is further aided in its movement by a pumping mechanism made up of the alternating pressures, which are created between the chest cavity and the abdominal cavity, as we breathe. This action is accompanied by an up and down movement of the main dividing feature between the chest and the abdomen, the diaphragm.

Thus, if there is poor muscular activity, and shallow breathing, there is likely to be a degree of 'pooling' in the veinous system. This can result in a degree of back pressure building up, affecting the arterial system, and thus creating a need for higher pressure from the heart as it beats, or from the muscular coating of the arterial system. This increases the internal pressure of the arteries, and possibly of the heart itself.

Thus on a purely mechanical level it is possible for the

blood-pressure to be increased through lack of use of the body, and inadequate breathing. Conversely exercise and proper breathing aid high blood-pressure. We will look more closely at exercise and breathing later in the book.

Low Blood-Pressure

Blood-pressure is vital to life. High blood-pressure is a threat to it. There is of course a condition called low blood-pressure as well, and we should be aware of its implications. Low blood-pressure, or hypotension, is said to exist if an adult has a systolic pressure which is persistently below between 90 and 100mm/Hg. It is usually accompanied by a pulse rate which is rapid but weak, and which will alter, by a reduction of as much as 40 beats per minute, when the individual lies down. There may be no obvious symptoms, but more usually there is a feeling of lassitude, giddiness (especially when standing from the sitting position) and a muzzy head. Fainting may occur at such times. This may in fact be an inherited constitutional state, or it may be the result of any of a number of pathological processes, such as some forms of heart disease, kidney problems, malnutrition, tuberculosis, haemorrhage or physical and mental exhaustion.

The treatment depends upon the cause, of course, but obvious irritants such as the use of purgatives, very hot baths, and excessive prolonged standing should be avoided. The condition is helped by general exercise, and abdominal exercise, or support.

As will become clear the passage of blood returning to the heart can be severely compromised by a number of conditions involving the abdominal area, for example pregnancy, or constipation, can send the pressure up, and weak muscular support can cause it to drop. Thus, in low blood-pressure from whatever cause the abdominal musculature and breathing mechanism can be used to great effect in assisting the return of blood to the heart. Awareness of low blood-pressure as a possible factor in conditions in which there is a feeling of weakness, exhaustion and lightheadedness can be useful in pointing to such simple methods of correction.

Breathing function and abdominal tone are of importance in high blood-pressure as well, as we will see in the chapters dealing with practical self-help methods of coping with hypertension.

Before continuing to look at the implications of high blood-pressure, and a variety of causes for this, most of which lie within the control of the individual to alter, it will be as well to briefly look at a few of the other factors which can alter the pressure as the blood passes round the body. Anything which causes the blood-vessels, through which the blood is passing, to be constricted or narrowed will result in greater pressure being called for to push the blood through them. Thus a variety of factors which can cause increased tension or hardening of the muscular coating of the arteries and arterioles can be responsible, especially if this is a long term situation. Stress and tension are therefore seen as possible factors in raising pressure. If the arteries and arterioles become narrowed, because of deposits within them, then the same thing happens (arteriosclerosis or hardening of the arteries). Since the blood, returning to the heart, has to pass through the kidneys for filtering, the health of these vital organs can influence the pressure. The blood has also to pass through the liver, for detoxification and to collect vital nutrients, and so a similar problem can arise if there is less than a healthy liver to work with. Both the liver and the kidneys will be considered in more detail later.

It has been noted that many people have high blood-pressure associated with the use of salt, which can alter the biochemical balance in the bloodstream and the body as a whole. Sodium chloride (salt) can produce major imbalances in the biochemical constituency of the body fluids in general which can increase the degree of effort required by the heart to pump blood, thus raising pressure. As mentioned previously, anything which allows the venous blood to become sluggish in its return to the heart results in back-pressure on the arterial system also raising the pressure. Such factors as chronic constipation, abdominal tumours, pregnancy, poor muscular tone in the limbs and abdomen, combined with inadequate exercise, can all be contributors to such a state of affairs. Smoking can be a key factor in raising pressure by virtue of its action in constricting the small blood-vessels. The use of certain drugs (such as the Pill) can have a similar effect in sensitive individuals.

It is worth noting of course that we are all biologically and biochemically individual. Thus factors which affect one person may not affect another at all, or to the same degree. There are many people eating lashings of salt, and smoking heavily, with relatively normal blood-pressures (at least for the time being).

If we are to deal satisfactorily with an individuals' hypertension problems, then all major factors must be looked at, and those implicated as being possible causes should be dealt with, mainly by self-help methods. In this way the marvellous self-repairing mechanisms of the body can begin to restore normal function.

One of the most important causes of increased blood-pressure, which is frequently within our control, is overweight. For every pound of excess weight that is carried, there are a hundred miles of extra capillaries (tiny blood-vessels) for the heart to push blood through. The effect of being just a little overweight can therefore be a key factor, in the blood-pressure picture.

Some possible causes of high blood-pressure, as outlined above, will be more closely examined in the following chapters. First, however, we must look at the implications of high blood-pressure to see just what it can mean in terms of life and health.

1.

The Implications of High Blood-Pressure

High blood-pressure can be shown to reduce severely the life expectancy of the individual. A rise to a level of only 130/90mm/Hg, which until recently was thought to be so small a rise as to be unworthy of attention, is shown to cut male life expectancy (at age 35) by four years. A rise at that age, to a level of 140/95mm/Hg, knocks an estimated (by the Society of Actuaries) nine years off life expectancy.

By the time blood-pressure has reached a level of 150/100mm/ Hg at age 35, a not uncommon level in modern life, the reduction in anticipated life is over sixteen years. Not only this, but the quality of that life can be severely disrupted and lowered, because of the increased risk of becoming an invalid for many of those remaining years due to coronary heart disease, or stroke, or congestive heart failure.

In long term studies conducted in America it was shown that the risks of one or other of these disasters occurring is often trebled when blood-pressure rises above normal. In the case of congestive heart failure the risk is quadrupled.

Every possible factor, in causing such a rise, is therefore of the greatest importance since, as will be seen, many of the causes are capable of being eliminated from the scene, and the condition can thus frequently be restored to a close approximation of normality.

Since there is no single, clear cut cause of high blood-pressure, there can be no standardized form of therapy. The total combined history of stresses, inherited factors, dietary indiscretions and lifestyle all combine to interact with the particular physiology and psychology of the individual, creating a situation in which the body may have to attempt to maintain circulatory function by means of raising the blood-pressure. A drug prescribed to counteract this would either aim at fluid elimination by increasing the kidney output (i.e. a diuretic drug) or it might attempt to expand the contracted blood vessel (i.e. a vasodilatory drug), thus reducing the effort of the heart in pumping the blood through the vessels.

These are symptom-orientated methods. They see the high blood-pressure as the entity that requires altering. The drug may well succeed in altering the situation, by lowering the pressure. This, though, would not necessarily be either desirable or scientifically acceptable, since all that would have been achieved would be to have left the underlying causes unchanged. The issue is not whether blood-pressure can be speedily lowered by drug methods, for often it can, but whether this is the correct way of approaching a complex problem.

If there is fluid retention, is it not more appropriate to remove the reasons for this? A natural, non-drug, programme will do this in many cases, and will bring with it all sorts of additional health bonuses. The drug approach not only does nothing for the underlying causes, but brings with it inevitable side-effects, some of which are potentially very dangerous.

What Affects Blood-Pressure?

Blood-pressure is the force exerted by the blood, within the arteries. It depends upon a number of interacting variables, such as the force of the heart beat, the elasticity of the blood-vessel walls; the resistance, or back-pressure, from the body as a whole (such factors as fluid levels, and weight influence this); as well as the degree of muscular pressure on the small blood-vessels; the viscosity (thickness) of the blood, and its total volume. All these factors have an effect upon the pressure, as do the relative health and efficiency of the liver and kidneys, and the tone and efficiency of the muscular and respiratory (breathing) systems of the body. There are many ways in which a combination of these factors can create a situation which calls for the body to raise the pressure abnormally, and we can frequently normalize the situation by our own efforts, by removing causative factors.

There are also many situations in which blood-pressure may rise, and yet not be significant, or be cause for concern. It is not uncommon, for example, for the more easily influenced aspect of the blood-pressure (systolic blood-pressure) to be raised, under upsetting or stressful conditions. This is not considered of any great importance, as long as the other part of the blood-pressure remains relatively normal (the diastolic pressure). In some people there is a tendency for the pressure to rise quite rapidly, but it settles towards normal just as fast. This is of interest, but not of great significance. The critical influence which high blood-pressure can have on the health of the individual is now much more clearly understood.

It used to be thought that blood-pressure necessarily rose with age. In fact it was commonly held that the systolic pressure ought to be somewhere around a figure of 100 plus the age of the individual. This is now known to be totally inaccurate, since blood-pressure ought not vary greatly with age, and when it does, it is no more than evidence of the effects of those aspects of life which mitigate against the pressure reading remaining at a normal level.

In societies in which diet has remained relatively unaffected by modern trends, and in which an unpolluted and peaceful existence has been maintained, blood-pressure remains at youthful levels into old age, and coronary disease is almost unknown. The blood-pressure level enjoyed in early adult life, if health is normal, is the level which is ideal throughout life. The average desirable levels are thought to be in the region of 120 systolic and 80 diastolic, and anything in excess of this is thought to be undesirable. Dangerous implications are considered possible if the pressure is over 160 systolic or 95 diastolic. Levels between the desired 120/80 and the dangerous 160/95 are of importance as they indicate that there is a trend away from normal towards danger, and that action is called for.

Hypertension
Hypertension is the leading physiological abnormality contributing towards death in Western society. In the

UK it is the major contributory factor in heart disease and strokes, which together comprise by far the greatest causes of death. The sad fact is that most people suffering from high blood-pressure do not know it, and the longer the condition remains undiagnosed, the greater the chances of it causing damage. It is the lack of symptoms of an obvious nature which frequently prevents many people from being aware of their condition of high blood-pressure. It can, and often does, produce symptoms (see below) but more often than not these are absent, or so mild as to be taken as part of normal existence. In some people blood-pressure fluctuates dramatically depending upon such underlying factors as stress or food sensitivities. In most though, the pressure just gradually creeps upwards, unnoticed.

Some or all of the following symptoms may accompany hypertension:

> Ringing or buzzing in the ears, or a loudly audible pulsing in the head.
> Frequent nosebleeds.
> Dizziness, especially when altering position (although low blood-pressure may also be responsible).
> Headaches or a feeling of fullness in the head.
> Alterations in the heart rate, including palpitations.
> Frequency of urination.
> Swollen lower limbs.
> Unexplained irritability.
> Unexplained aches and pains.
> Unnatural tiredness.

It is just as likely, however, that none of the above will be noticed and that blood-pressure will be high without symptoms.

There are also, it should be noted, many people who are born with a natural tendency towards a higher blood-pressure than average. Family tendencies towards this are not uncommon and call for special attention to the problem.

The commonly held view that sodium, derived from salt, is a key to high blood-pressure is now known to be only part of the picture, and we will consider this in greater detail in a later chapter. What has emerged is that far from salt automatically sending blood-pressure up, it is the case that this happens only in those people born with a predisposition to high blood-pressure, who are also what is known as 'salt sensitive'. When such individuals are exposed to an average salt intake, they show signs of higher blood-pressure. Other individuals can apparently ingest larger amounts of salt without this effect. This illustrates the genetic or inborn nature of hypertension in many people, and shows that simplistic solutions, such as everyone cutting down on salt, would be likely to achieve only partial success because a limited section of the public is salt sensitive with a predisposition towards high blood-pressure.

Once high blood-pressure is a fact, the amount of damage that can result will also vary considerably from person to person. Many other factors, some inborn, some acquired, will decide just who will succumb to coronary disease or stroke, or who will indeed survive to old age in apparent good health despite hypertension. This is not in any way meant to suggest that hypertension should be ignored, only that its effects will not be uniformly harmful. In the main it is safe to say that health will be better if pressure is low or normal, rather than if it is high. Statistically, life expectancy is greater, and levels of well-being into old age are better if pressure is normal.

It is important for blood-pressure to be monitored at regular intervals, especially if there is any family history of cardiovascular disease or of high blood-pressure. This can be done by regular visits to a health professional, or by the use of simple self-monitoring equipment which is now available at relatively low cost.

Since high blood-pressure is a potential risk to life itself, and since it is also, as we will see, relatively easy in most cases to control by self-help methods, there is every reason for paying attention to this vital health indicator. This does not mean becoming obsessed with health matters, but that, at regular intervals, say once every six months, blood-pressure should be checked. It is a legitimate question to ask whether there is any need for self-help, since there are a variety of drugs available which can control hypertension. There is no doubt that under certain conditions anti-hypertensive drugs are called for, especially in short-term use, if the pressure is dangerously high. However, there is abundant evidence that all such drugs have side-effects (see next chapter), some very serious, and that blood-pressure is controllable by safe non-drug methods, in the majority of cases. Such non-drug methods may well also bring many other health benefits with them, as well as being infinitely satisfying by virtue of the knowledge that the condition has been dealt with personally, and that causes have been tackled rather than symptoms alone.

Many esteemed medical authorities have come to the view that drug therapy for hypertension is at best of short term value, and that the type of measures that will be presented in subsequent chapters offer a far more scientific and acceptable alternative. This is because of growing evidence that drug control of hypertension, whilst apparently effective in achieving symptomatic control, has little overall benefit in terms of increasing life-expectancy or in preventing ultimate cardiovascular disease from emerging. In contrast, lifestyle and dietary alterations, together with behavioural reforms which combine to lower high blood-pressure, confer distinct benefits to the individual in regard to life-expectancy, as well as health levels being enhanced. This then is not so much a way of avoiding drugs for no good reason, but of a better, safer, and more efficient way of dealing with a major health problem.

If you wish to avoid cardiovascular disease, heart attacks, thrombosis, strokes, angina and myriad other possible complications of hypertension, then the advice contained in the following chapters should be studied, understood and applied.

Areas of importance to which we must apply ourselves are those which explain just how different factors can produce high blood-pressure. After that we will be ready to look at methods of avoiding these occurrences and of dealing with existing hypertension.

2.

Blood-Pressure Variations

There are a number of important clues that we can obtain from blood-pressure readings which can tell us much about the general function of the body and its health status.

For example, if we wish to establish what is known as the 'work-load' of the heart, we can do a simple sum in which we multiply the pulse rate (number of beats of the heart per minute) by the systolic blood-pressure (the higher of the two figures taken). The normal figure resulting from such a sum would range between 8000 and 9500. Should it amount to something in excess of 9500, then there is a chance of problems arising in either the kidneys or the liver, or there may be athero-sclerotic developments (fatty deposits building up on the inside of blood-vessels which restrict blood flow), and further investigation is called for. If however the total arrived at is below 8000, then there is a chance of either what is called 'adrenal insufficiency' (in which the hormonal production of the adrenal glands is under par for some reason) or there may be a degree of nutritional deficiency or generalized weakness. These would require investigation, and could probably be dealt with nutritionally. So the 'work-load' represents just how hard the heart has to work, being the product of the number of times it beats multiplied by the force with which it beats.

It is possible to obtain further information from the blood-pressure reading about the status of the adrenal glands (which produce that most important hormone adrenaline). This involves having the blood-pressure taken when lying down (after being in that position for at least four minutes) and then immediately after standing up. There should be a rise in the systolic pressure of at least 5mm/Hg on standing. If not, then the adrenal glands are considered to be weak, under strain, or depleted, and action is called for to restore them to normal. This involves stress reduction, adequate exercise and rest, and nutrient support as outlined in later chapters, as well as the avoidance of stimulants such as drugs, coffee, alcohol and cigarettes.

If the diastolic blood-pressure (the lower of the two figures) is consistently higher than 95, then there is a strong suspicion of problems relating to either the liver (the body's main organ of detoxification) or the kidneys, and further investigation is called for.

Testing for High Blood-Pressure

There are simple home tests which can be carried out to assess whether there is a potential for the development of high blood-pressure as a result of back-pressure on the venous system. This can also be taken, to some extent, as an indication of the current efficiency of liver function, at least as far as any influence it has on the circulating blood.

With the balls of the thumbs, press down on a fleshy part of the legs (or chest, or between the shoulder blades, if you are testing someone else) for about five seconds. The pressure should not be heavy but of medium intensity (enough to cause discomfort but not pain if you were using that amount of pressure on the closed eyes). Release the pressure, and if a blanched, white area remains visible, it indicates that increased vein pressure exists. Normal vein pressure would not allow a white area to remain. Such venous back-pressure can result from a sequence of events which can include either the liver or the kidneys being unable to handle adequately the filtering of blood that passes through them. This can eventually result in extra effort being required from the heart muscle. Back-pressure can also impair circulation to, and through, these vital organs, themselves causing increased problems.

The elevation of blood-pressure, via this type of sequence is therefore a secondary event, following on from original problems in the major organs involved. Evidence of such back-pressure, in someone with no evidence of high blood-pressure, can be taken as an indication of problems as yet in their early stages. Attention to the basic requirements of the body, in terms of diet and exercise, and stress reduction, will go a long way to minimizing the likelihood of further degenerative, or pathological changes.

In medical terminology the following are the actual definitions of different levels of blood-pressure.

If the diastolic pressure reading is 85mm/Hg or lower, then it is classified as 'Normal'. Between 85 and

89mm/Hg it is classified as 'High Normal Blood-Pressure'. Between 90 and 104mm/Hg it is classified as 'Mild Hypertension'. From 105 to 114mm/Hg it is classified as 'Moderate Hypertension'. Above 114mm/Hg is classified as 'Severe Hypertension'.

The systolic reading is regarded as 'Normal' if it is less than 140mm/Hg (assuming the diastolic pressure to be normal). If it is between 140 and 159mm/Hg, then it is classified as 'Borderline Isolated Systolic Hypertension'; and if greater than that as 'Isolated Systolic Hypertension'.

When the pressure is between 90 and 104mm/Hg diastolic, and/or 140 and 199mm/Hg systolic, there is a need to recheck the pressure at least every two months. If diastolic pressure exceeds 105mm/Hg and/or the systolic exceeds 200mm/hg, then detailed and speedy evaluation of the condition is called for by a medical or naturopathic practitioner.

Note: The advice contained in this book can be applied to the prevention of hypertension, or to the treatment of any stage of hypertension. However, should the diastolic pressure exceed 105mm/Hg, and/or the systolic exceed 200mm/Hg, then the methods outlined should be combined with advice and/or treatment from a qualified practitioner.

Should drugs be employed in the treatment of high blood-pressure they may fall into one of the following categories (a combination is usual).

Diuretics

These speed the elimination of fluid from the body. They are known in many cases to cause raised cholesterol levels, glucose intolerance, sexual dysfunction, and to unbalance the potassium levels in the body, as some of their side-effects. The potassium loss caused by these drugs is usually balanced by taking extra supplements of this vital substance.

Adrenergic Antagonists

These are a range of drugs which act in a variety of ways to influence the function of adrenaline, thus influencing circulation and blood-pressure. Among their many side-effects are: headaches, palpitations, weakness, dry mouth, asthma, bizarre dreams, fatigue, insomnia, sexual dysfunction, cholesterol levels raised, or lowered levels of the beneficial aspect of cholesterol (high density lipoprotein). Low blood-pressure can result from some forms of adrenergic antagonists, and in general great care has to be taken by monitoring the use of these drugs.

Vasodilators

These drugs relax the controls that cause pressure to be exerted on the blood-vessel walls, thus allowing them to expand, so that less effort is needed from the heart to push blood through them. Side-effects can include rapid heart beat, headache, rashes, etc.

Other drugs to lower blood-pressure include those that act on certain enzyme systems, and on calcium metabolism. A similar list of symptoms and precautionary warnings are found with these drugs. Altogether the field of drug therapy for high blood-pressure is littered with the names of once popular drugs which have been withdrawn as a result of unacceptable side-effects. This is not really surprising, since the aim of each of these drugs, in its own way, is to alter one or other aspect of the complicated circulatory system, with a view to lowering the blood-pressure. Whilst frequently achieving that goal, there is in each and every case a degree of side-effect apparent as the system tries to cope with the alterations forced upon it by the drug. The very nature of high blood-pressure makes it likely that anything forcefully altering aspects of the body's physiology, is bound to have repercussions throughout the body.

Blood-pressure is a function. High blood-pressure is a function which is exaggerated as the system attempts to cope with unusual or undesirable factors. To alter, using drugs, the blood-pressure, without in some way attempting to deal with the causes of its elevation, is to court disaster. This is not to say that, in extreme cases, there is not a good case for the employment of one or other of these drugs, at least in the short-term. This does not in any way excuse the avoidance of dealing with causes which must precede any real control or return to normality of a blood-pressure which is high. There is a growing awareness, amongst medical researchers and practitioners, of the need for greater attention to causative factors, as well as to non-pharmacological methods such as those outlined in this book. These include weight reduction, salt limitation, stress reduction methods, moderation of alcohol and tobacco usage, exercise, behaviour modification, and dietary changes. The attitude to these methods seems to be that whilst they hold great promise, and should be used whenever appropriate, they do not take the place of drug control. This may be a fair comment where pressure is so high that it endangers life. Combining drug treatment with a non-drug, self-help approach, would then seem to be the best choice. In the field of prevention and dealing with mild hypertension, the non-drug methods must be seen as superior, since they deal with causes, not symptoms, and they are without exception, safe.

No advice contained in this book should be taken as advice to avoid medical care. Awareness of alternatives, and of the inherent dangers in drug methods, should lead to an intelligent and co-operative involvement in the programme to recover and to maintain health at its optimum level, as well as preventing ill health, including high blood-pressure.

We will now examine more closely some of the major causes of hypertension.

3.

The Causes of High Blood-Pressure

Stress
This is probably the most easily demonstrated cause of increasing blood-pressure. Whenever we are under stress, upset, angry, anxious, or called upon to adapt to unusual conditions or situations, the body responds by preparing for activity by co-ordinating a variety of rapid internal changes. Among the most important of the changes which take place almost instantaneously after any such challenge, is the release of the hormone adrenaline by glands which lie above the kidneys. This, and other secretions, cause the blood-vessels to narrow, aiding in the rapid transmission of oxygenated blood to the muscles and brain. This is also achieved by increasing the heart rate and, naturally enough, by a rise in blood-pressure. Arousal of this sort is a normal physiological response to the demands of life. Unfortunately though, in modern life, such demands can become repetitive or even constant. In such a situation the rise in blood-pressure and the narrowing in diameter of the blood-vessels, can also be almost a constant factor. If blood-pressure is already higher than normal, then such

additional increases can be severely compromising for the body, and can result in a cerebral accident (stroke) due to a failure of one of the blood-vessels to cope with the increased strain of high-pressure. In any case, the rise in blood-pressure, via stress factors, can be seen to be a major cause of chronic hypertension.

Learning to avoid arousal, anger, anxiety and other forms of obvious emotional stress, is therefore of some importance to anyone repetitively affected in this way. The application of de-stressing methods, including relaxation and meditation techniques, or of bio-feedback methods, is often helpful, and this will be discussed in later chapters. It should be clear though, that each individual cause of high blood-pressure is seldom found to be acting alone, and more commonly there will be a number of interacting elements making up the complex picture.

Salt
Salt may be one such additional factor. This has been shown in many individuals to have the ability to upset the delicate biochemical balance that exists in the body between sodium (a constituent of salt) and potassium. It is known that in areas of the world where salt intake is high, there is also a tendency for high blood-pressure to be prevalent. Among many population groups where the salt intake is below 500mg a day, there is often a tendency for blood-pressure to fall rather than rise with advancing age. The converse has also been noted. Indeed, in one group of South Sea Islanders, who cook their vegetables in sea water, and ingest as much as 15,000mg of salt daily, the blood-pressure of all people, including children, was elevated.

There is, however, known to be a degree of individual susceptibility. This susceptibility is also known to be greater in young people, so that a high salt habit, started in infancy, may be seen to be laying the foundation for high blood-pressure in later life. Although subsequent restriction of salt is seldom enough to return blood-pressure to normal, it does improve the picture to some extent. It seems that high intakes of sodium, in salt, has a depressing effect upon potassium levels. These two minerals interact in a close manner in the transport of nutrients to the cells, and the discharge of wastes from the cells. Anything which dramatically alters the relationship between them, also alters the dynamics of cellular physiology with grave repercussions. A tendency can develop for extra-cellular fluid to build up, and this manifests itself, in the body generally, as swollen areas. This creates an extra degree of pressure on the tiny blood-vessels and thus influences blood-pressure as a whole. The usual medical treatment of such a situation is to use diuretics which will 'flush' extra fluid from the body via the kidneys. This is at best a short term measure since it does nothing to alter the reasons for the imbalance (although most diuretics are given additional potassium to prevent further imbalance).

The prevention of high blood-pressure would therefore seem to call for the avoidance of a high salt intake in infancy, and the moderation of its use generally. This is the safest advice, since although some people can obviously eat salt with impunity, there is no way of knowing who this applies to until evidence of its harmlessness in the body is deduced by the maintenance of normal blood-pressure into old age. Cutting down salt in existing cases of hypertension can certainly help to mitigate against the condition getting worse, and can help in reduction of excessive levels. However, on its own, salt reduction will seldom allow a return to normal pressure. It should be seen as just one of a number of interconnecting factors in a programme to restore normality.

Smoking

Smoking is another common habit which has a direct and often dramatic, effect upon blood-pressure. The systolic pressure can rise by as much as 25mm/Hg within seconds of the first puff of a cigarette (or pipe, or cigar). Once again this is because of the production by the body of adrenaline, and as in the stress example, discussed above, the repetitive nature of the insult is what causes progressive damage. Any smoker will notice that, in time, the circulation to the extremities will become impaired, and cold hands and feet will be common. This is evidence of the restricting effect upon the blood-vessels, and the obvious result of this is to send blood-pressure upwards as the body fights to get blood through narrower channels. Often such narrowing can lead to complete obliteration of the circulation to a limb, and the result of this may be gangrene, and amputation.

In less dramatic ways the average smoker can destroy normal function and increase blood-pressure steadily over a long period of time. The combination of a highly stressed individual who also smokes, can be seen to be a prototype for the hypertensive individual who is a candidate for an early coronary or stroke. Both factors, stress and smoking, are capable of being altered and the condition normalized, thus avoiding the ultimate disaster.

Eating Meat

Eating meat has been shown to increase blood-pressure. Approximately one hundred confirmed adult vegetarians were compared with a matched group of non-vegetarians living in the same urban environment. The average blood-pressure of the vegetarians was 126/77mm/Hg, and that of the meat eaters 147/88. There was a significantly lower blood-pressure in all age groups in the vegetarian group, and only two per cent of the vegetarians had high blood-pressure (over 160/95) as compared with 26 per cent of the meat eating group. The family history of high blood-pressure was similar in both groups, and weight similarity was taken into account in all comparisons. The main difference between the groups, as far as individual nutrients were concerned, was found to be much higher intake of potassium amongst the vegetarians which is thought to be the significant factor in maintaining a lower blood-pressure amongst these individuals.

The vegetarians' diet was free of all meat and fish, and there were no more than three eggs eaten weekly, and hardly any dairy produce. The average pattern of eating was as follows:

Breakfast: Bread, fresh vegetables, yogurt or rice porridge.
Lunch: Vegetable salad, boiled vegetables including potatoes or rice, pastries and fruits.

Supper: Fresh vegetable salad with almonds, peanuts or nuts and fruit.

The fact that a sodium/potassium imbalance, resulting from a high salt intake can result in high blood-pressure, and that a diet rich in potassium apparently has the opposite effect, gives us a clue as to the type of dietary pattern that would be helpful in both preventing and correcting high blood-pressure.

Hardening of the Arteries: Also known as arteriosclerosis, this is the condition which many see as the main cause of chronic hypertension. When the arteries become narrowed by the deposition on their walls of substances such as calcium, cholesterol, fibrin, etc. (known collectively as atheroma), the passage for blood becomes gradually reduced, and the consequences are grave. Among the early symptoms is a rise in blood-pressure to overcome the narrowed diameter of the arteries. This condition, which can itself be the major cause of further problems, is not able to simply arise in the body without predisposing causes. So although arteriosclerosis is a cause of high blood-pressure, it is itself the result of biochemical alterations which may be the result of nutritional imbalances and deficiencies. It is obviously justifiable, and often essential, to tackle the existing concretions in the arteries by using a variety of means, some of which we will discuss, however the prevention of the condition is infinitely preferable. One of the major causes of arterial damage of this kind is the activity in the body of a minute structure called a 'free radical'.

Free Radicals Explained: These are fragments of atoms or molecules which are created in the body in a cellular situation in which there is inadequate oxygen. The fragment is possessed of an unpaired free electron which allows the free radical to attach itself to an electron from any passing cell. This can start a chain reaction, because the particle which has lost its electron automatically attempts to balance the situation by capturing the first available electron it comes across. Thus the free radical can be seen to be a highly reactive and disruptive factor.

Its life may pass in a matter of a few thousandths of a second, and yet the chain reaction it initiates may have vast repurcussions involving many thousands of cells and molecules. Should such a reaction take place in an artery, then the resulting damage would affect the cells lining the walls of that artery. Cells in the artery wall can be induced, in this manner, to mutate, and this in turn results in the deposition in the damaged area of plaque, which is made of fibrin (blood protein laid down as a protective blanket) and also undesirable superfluous fats which may be present in the blood stream, such as cholesterol, triglycerides and also calcium. Thus one cause of the formation of atheroma, and consequent narrowing and hardening of the arteries, is the free radical. Predisposition towards free radical damage may include a lack of antioxidant substances, which mop up and destroy free radicals before they can do any damage. These include vitamins C and E, as well as minerals such as zinc and selenium. There are also a number of amino acids which have this function, including methionine, cysteine and glutathione peroxidase. Vitamins B_1, B_5 and B_6 are also of assistance in controlling free radical activity. When there is a relative lack of such nutrients, and the body is exposed to pollution (cigarette smoke, alcohol, environmental pollution, etc.) or a diet high in factors which can degrade and form free radicals, such as fats and oils, then the formation of these substances becomes more likely.

High-fibre foods are one way of ensuring that free radical production is reduced, since this type of food removes superfluous fats from the system. Much free radical activity begins with the breakdown products of foods in the bowel. The amount of time food residues spend in the bowel is important in this regard, since in the average Western bowel the transit time for food is between 75 and 100 hours, whereas the more primitive, high fibre diet of less sophisticated cultures produces a transit time of about 35 hours with less, if any, free radical activity, and no atherosclerosis. This is also a key factor in the prevention of some major forms of cancer. If we consider that the major demonstrable alteration leading to high blood-pressure and heart disease is a degeneration of the arteries which carry fresh blood to the body as a whole and to the heart muscle itself, then the importance of free radical activity becomes clearer, as do the aspects of life which are conducive to free radical activity. These include a diet inadequate in essential antioxidant substances such as vitamins C, E, A, B_1, B_5, B_6, zinc, selenium, etc. as well as a diet rich in fats, and an environment which contains pollutants and irritants such as smoke and alcohol (in excess).

Other Factors Contributing to Arteriosclerosis: There

are a number of other identifiable factors which can be major contributors to the development of arterial plaque deposits. One of these is chromium deficiency. Chromium is an important part of what is known as the Glucose Tolerance Factor (GTF). This is necessary for the production, and use by the body, of insulin, which controls the levels of sugar in the blood. If dietary chromium is low, and it usually is on a Western diet rich in refined carbohydrate products, then arteriosclerosis appears to develop more rapidly. The precise relationship is not yet clear, but the fact is that there is a demonstrable lack of chromium in individuals who die of coronary disease. The best sources of chromium are from yeast and black pepper.

Dietary Fats: Cholesterol is a vital part of the body economy, and 90 per cent of it is manufactured by the body itself. It is made in the liver and digestive tract from such food elements as sugars, proteins and fats. The 10 per cent of cholesterol in the body that is derived directly from the diet is therefore not the most important element in the situation. However, if there is a high cholesterol level (and this is undesirable) then as well as finding ways of reducing the levels in the body, there should be some control over the intake of cholesterol-rich foods. The dietary pattern suggested later in the book will take care of both aspects of this requirement.

It is worth noting that cholesterol comprises a number of constituents, one of which, high density lipoprotein (HDL), is in fact extremely beneficial. It acts as a scavenger of unwanted substances in the arteries and helps protect against heart disease. Not everyone has high levels of HDL in their cholesterol, indeed some have an excess of low density lipoprotein (LDL) instead. Interestingly one research finding has been that a moderate amount of alcohol intake (1 ½ glasses of wine daily) increases a certain form of HDL and this may act to protect against heart disease. Higher intakes of alcohol however are known to be harmful, leading to liver damage as well as an increased risk of other degenerative diseases. The aim of a diet which wishes to reduce the dangers of arterial damage, and so reduce the risk of heart disease and high blood-pressure, must be to lower overall cholesterol levels to safe limits, at the same time as increasing the proportion of HDL in that which remains. It is also interesting to note that in young men, between 16 and 27, the severe cystic form of acne which sometimes manifests itself, is associated with a low level of HDL, and that this can be seen as an early warning of cardiac problems to follow.

The process of damage to the arteries passes from the original free radical lesion, through the laying down of fibrin and the collection in the area of excess cholesterol and other blood fats to a final stage in which calcification of the lesion begins. This involves the linking of the cholesterol deposits with calcium, in an electrically charged attraction, which bonds like concrete. More fatty materials and calcium continue to build onto this structure, making the artery more rigid and narrower and consequently limiting the passage of blood and raising the blood-pressure as a consequence.

Bypass Surgery? When the blood-vessels which carry freshly oxygenated blood from the lungs to the heart muscles become affected by this process, then the heart is in danger of oxygen starvation, and of a heart attack. This occurs when, through the narrowing process, the heart becomes starved of oxygen and some of it actually dies (necrosis); or else a fragment of the atheromatous plaque breaks off and blocks the artery. By this time the individual will probably have had symptoms of angina (pain on exertion) for some time, as well as breathlessness. The current surgical procedure is to remove blood-vessels from one of the limbs and graft these onto the heart so that they bypass the blocked arteries and carry fresh blood to the heart muscle. Bypass surgery has become a major industry (an estimated three billion dollars a year in the USA). The results can be dramatic. However in many cases the benefits are short lived, and fifty per cent of these patients are dead within three years. The majority of the others are showing signs of silting up the new arteries by then, and the long term prospects are not good. This is largely because of the failure of the individual to reform those aspects of their life which contributed to the problem in the first place.

An alternative method to surgery is being used by certain pioneering clinics in the USA, this is called chelation therapy. This involves the use of a substance to remove from the arteries the calcified material which has obstructed them. It is accompanied by a programme of reformed nutrition to prevent recurrence. The decalcification of the arteries lowers blood-pressure as it removes one of reasons for its increase. There are also a variety of natural methods of chelating calcium from the blood-vessels, and these will be outlined later (see oral chelation page 84).

The dietary and exercise programme which will

prevent, and help to cope with high blood-pressure will also be outlined later, but at this stage it is important to realize that most of the factors which lead to the degeneration of the cardiovascular system, apart from inherited factors, lie firmly in the control of the individual. Some of the inherited factors can also be influenced, for example deficiency of vitamin B_6 in a pregnant mother can result in early changes to the blood vessels of her child, which can lead to athero-sclerosis later.

Among the chronic health problems which can, over a period of time, result in the development of high blood-pressure, are conditions involving the kidneys and liver. As blood is obliged to pass through these organs on its circuit of the body, any of a wide range of ailments affecting them can influence the pressure. It is not within the scope of this book to look comprehensively at all these possible conditions however, it should be clear that if there is a major problem involving the kidneys or liver then expert advice is required. If the general advice regarding nutrition, stress reduction and exercise is followed, then any tendency for minor dysfunction of the liver in particular, should be eliminated. Kidney function will also be improved by following the same advice but may require more specialized individual attention.

The liver is an organ which is easily affected by a less than adequate diet, especially one which includes excessive fats and refined foods, together with stimulants such as coffee, tea and alcohol. The reforms outlined in Chapter 5 together with periodic detoxifi-cation via fasting (see Chapter 6) will enable it to regenerate quite remarkably. There are also a number of specific aids that can be employed, such as amino acids, to speed detoxification of this most important organ. Some experts believe that general liver congestion resulting from nutritional imbalance and lack of exercise, is one of the main reasons for high blood-pressure.

The drinking of tap water, especially in cities and industrialized areas, is thought to produce additional strain for the kidneys due to the content of undesirable chemicals and contaminants. The use of a water filter on taps, or the substitution of spring or mineral water for tap water, is an alternative. Perhaps the best water of all is that derived from the cooking of vegetables. Once water has been boiled, chlorine, one of the harmful factors in tap water, will have been eliminated. The mineral content of water in which vegetables have been cooked is high. This has been called potassium broth, and it will be referred to in the chapter dealing with suggested foods. A fast on such a broth, or its use in regular eating patterns, is most valuable. It helps to balance the sodium-potassium ratio which, as we have seen, can be a cause of high blood-pressure.

Some individuals also display calcium imbalance which can be related to kidney problems. It is frequently found that an increased intake of calcium and vitamin C helps in the normalization of such problems. Such an imbalance may be accompanied by night-time cramps. Advice on quantities of supplements will be given later. A connection has also been established between a dangerous form of hypertension which occurs in late pregnancy and calcium deficiency. The toxaemia of pregnancy includes high blood-pressure as one of its symptoms. The addition of half a gram of calcium daily reduces the chances of this happening. Zinc is also often deficient in such conditions, and experts believe that this is linked to the calcium deficiency.

The interaction of many substances can be seen to be important, and this gives a clear indication that a balanced wholefood diet containing adequate quantities of all the vital nutrients is important, especially to the expectant mother. If these nutrients are unavailable through diet alone, then supplements can be used. In general terms high blood-pressure usually results from a combination of stress factors, inadequate exercise and nutritional imbalance. The many ways in which different levels of these factors can manifest themselves in a variety of health problems, including high blood-pressure, is evidence of the complexity of the human body.

Hypertension may result from different causes and so the approach to its normalization must vary. Similar causative factors in different people may result in different ailments. Generalization as to what will result from particular habits is unwise. A high salt diet, with a highly stressed lifestyle may produce quite different health problems in different individuals, whereas apparently identical symptom patterns may have quite different causes.

In order to correct the dietary pattern towards normal, general trends requires analysis; similarly with stress patterns and lifestyle habits. The following sets of questions will help you to do this. You are unique, and the pattern you require to help towards a normal healthy pattern is also personally unique to you. The broad pattern of our needs may be the same, but idiosyncratic requirements, which all of us have, require attention for the achievement of optimum health.

4.

Assessing Your Dietary and Lifestyle Pattern

Nutritional Checklist
The aim of this series of questions is to assess your general awareness and implementation of the importance of correct nutritional practices. The more 'Yes' answers in the first set of questions the more need to reform your overall pattern of eating. The ideal would be for all these answers to be 'No', but this is unlikely. Answer 'Yes', 'No' or 'Sometimes' (where 'Sometimes' means not more than once a week, and 'No' means less than once a week. 'Yes' indicates about four times weekly, or more). Two 'Sometimes' answers can be taken to indicate a 'Yes' in totalling up your score at the end.

Do you eat refined (i.e. white) flour products?

Do you include sugar (any type) in your diet, or eat sweets?

Do you drink coffee, tea, chocolate or cola drinks?

Do you drink alcohol other than the equivalent of 1½ glasses of wine, or a pint of beer daily?

Do you eat foods containing any chemical additives (colouring, flavouring, etc.)?

Do you skip meals?

Do you pick at food between meals?

Do you eat more than 6oz (175g) of animal protein daily?

Do you eat convenience, ready-made foods e.g. instant mashed potatoes, T.V. dinners or tinned foods?

Do you add salt to your food?

Do you eat fried or highly seasoned and spiced foods?

Do you eat fatty meats, smoked or preserved foods?

The next series of questions should ideally all be answered 'Yes'. Use the same method of 'Yes', 'No' or 'Sometimes' in answering these.

Do you eat fresh fruit?

Do you eat salad?

Do you insist on fresh vegetables only? (not frozen or canned)

Do you use herbs or garlic for flavouring food?

Do you ensure adequate fibre in your diet?

Do you eat whole cereal products (such as brown rice and wholemeal bread)?

Do you drink bottled rather than chlorinated tap waters?

Do you take a multivitamin, or multimineral, supplement or a vitamin C tablet?

Do you eat non-animal proteins such as seeds, nuts, pulses?

Do you eat breakfast?

Do you eat natural yogurt?

Do you believe that what you eat affects your health in a major way for good or ill?

Score two points for each 'Yes', and one for each 'Sometimes'. Deduct the score of the second twelve questions, from the score of the first. An ideal total should be a minus number, or zero. Any score above zero indicates a need for reform, and if above 6 there is great need for attention to your diet. The methods outlined in later chapters on dietary changes should be studied and followed, and the target should be to work towards 12 'No' answers in the first set of questions, and 12 'Yes' answers in the second set when you retest yourself a few months hence.

Deficiencies
Deficiencies can be a major factor in allowing a decline in health which may accompany the onset of high blood-pressure, or cardiovascular problems. Answer the following questions. All of them can be the result of vitamin, mineral, enzyme or amino acid deficiency. They can have other causes, but if there are a number of 'Yes' answers, then following the programme of dietary changes given in this book, as well as adjusting your pattern to meet the requirements as outlined by the

previous two series of questions, will result in a great improvement.

Are your nails ridged?

Do your nails break easily?

Do you have white flecks in your nails?

Do your gums bleed when you clean your teeth?

Do you get frequent mouth ulcers?

Do you have stretch marks in your skin?

Do you get cracks in the corner of your mouth?

Does strong light irritate you?

Are your eyes, mouth or nose dry?

Have you lost your sense of taste or smell?

Does your skin scale or flake?

Do you have a strong body odour?

Do your feet smell strongly?

Do you bruise easily?

Do you have difficulty in recalling your dreams on waking?

Lifestyle
The pattern of life that we live is of major importance in normalizing tendencies towards hypertension caused by stress. The following series of questions should help to identify areas of your life which can be easily modified. The first six questions should yield a 'No' answer, and

the second six a 'Yes'. Modify accordingly to achieve this goal.

Do you work more than 5½ days weekly?

Do you work more than 10 hours on a work day?

Do you take less than half an hour for each main meal?

Do you eat quickly and not chew thoroughly?

Do you smoke?

Do you get less than seven hours sleep daily?

Do you regularly listen to relaxing music?

Do you practice daily relaxation or meditation?

Do you take thirty minutes exercise at least three times weekly?

Do you have a creative hobby (gardening, painting, needlework etc.)?

Do you play any non-competitive sport or activity such as walking, swimming or cycling or belong to a yoga or exercise class?

Do you try to have a siesta or short rest period during the day?

Do you have a regular massage, or osteopathic attention; or practise yoga or Tai Chi at home?

Do you spend at least half an hour outdoors, in daylight each day?

Hypertension Tendency
A tendency to high blood-pressure may exist as a result

of factors which may be elicited by the following series
of questions:

1. Were you raised, or do you live, in a city
   environment?

2. Were you *not* breast fed as a baby?

3. Are you showing any signs of premature ageing
   (early grey hair, early wrinkling, etc.)?

4. Have you been overweight, other than for brief
   periods (more than 15 per cent above ideal)?

5. Have you a history of following a strict low calorie
   diet?

6. Is there a family history of blood-pressure, heart
   disease or diabetes?

7. Have you been on the Pill for more than a two
   year period?

8. Do you eat meat daily?

9. Do you add salt to your food at table, or like salty
   cooked food?

10. Are you competitive, working to deadlines, easily
    irritated and/or ambitious?

If you are 50-60 years of age and your score in this last
series of questions is more than 4 'Yes' answers, then
you have a moderate tendency towards high blood-
pressure. If you are 60 years of age or more, and your
score is 3 or more 'Yes' answers, then the same applies.
If under fifty and 5 answers are 'Yes', then the same
applies. Higher scores increase the likelihood, lower

ones decrease it. This is a rough guide only, but is surprisingly accurate for most people.

The insights that this series of questions can give should help to focus your attention on those factors which are within your control. Some of course are not, for they are a matter of what has already happened. Overall though the majority of harmful influences that can mitigate towards high blood-pressure and cardiac problems lie well within your control. We will move on to self-help methods in the next chapter.

5.

Self-Help for High Blood-Pressure

In this section we are going to examine a variety of self-help methods which can be employed safely at home by anyone. It must be re-emphasized though that these recommendations are not meant to take the place of expert professional advice which should be sought if blood-pressure or health problems are anything other than mild. The methods presented all offer potential for general health improvement, and this is as it should be, since in the main, the advice is aimed at improving the total body-mind complex which makes up each of us.

By improving our general function and by avoiding those factors which specifically, or generally, create the situation in which high blood-pressure can manifest itself, the self-normalizing aspects of the body can come into play. This we call homoeostasis, a state which represents the body's constant striving for normality and health, which is continuous throughout life. We must replace bad habits with good ones; remove obstacles to health, and encourage the return to normality which will follow. Our attention will range through lifestyle and behaviour factors to exercise, breathing and relaxation methods, the use of nutritional supplements and dietary measures, all of which can be modified to help in the quest for health. Finally, we will examine the most ancient of therapeutic measures, fasting, as a means of self-help towards normal blood-pressure.

Lifestyle and Behaviour Factors

You will have answered the questions in the self-assessment chapter (page 53) and this will give a clear indication of those aspects of your lifestyle which need attention. Such simple measures as assuring that you get adequate rest and sleep, and that you modify any obvious stressful traits in the way you carry your everyday duties and activities, are all important.

We need adequate rest and sleep, and depending upon your particular needs this can mean anything from six to eight hours daily. If you have not been giving attention to this vital aspect of your life, begin now. An afternoon nap, or siesta, can also be a valuable aid. Many people find that this can be incorporated into their lunch break if they are at work. By having a twenty or thirty minute complete rest at this time of day, a good deal of stress can be eliminated, and the rest of the day can be faced with renewed energy. If longer is available, then an hour or so of actual sleep or just rest with the eyes closed, is ideal. Contrary to popular opinion this sort of rest does not subsequently interfere with the night's sleep, but has actually been shown to enhance it. It also helps considerably in the overall lowering of what has been called 'arousal', which simply means increased tension. If you can learn a simple relaxation method (see below) then this can be used at such a time to good effect.

This attention to adequate sleep and rest, should be accompanied by some thought as to general behaviour. If you are habitually in a hurry, always trying to do too many things, and often doing more than one thing at a time, then you may be what has been called a 'Type A' individual. This sort of person is often ambitious, competitive, quick moving, quick eating and quick talking. There is tendency to work to deadlines, and to be punctilious about time-keeping. Do you recognize any of your characteristics? The evidence is strong that this sort of personality is far more prone to cardio-vascular disease than the more relaxed, slow moving, 'Type B' personality. Many people have in fact, altered their behaviour from 'A' to 'B' by the simple expedient of concentrating on one aspect of behaviour at a time, say eating slowly, or being less anxious about time-keeping, with great success. Unfortunately the decision to attempt to alter behaviour is often not made until a serious scare, such as a coronary, has concentrated the minds of both the individual and his medical advisers. The preventative modification of such behaviour is obviously desirable, and this can have marked effect upon hypertension and general health. The adoption of creative, non-competitive hobbies, taking up regular, non-stressful exercise habits, preferably in the fresh air during daylight hours, as well as improving the sleep and rest factors discussed previously, all combine to create an atmosphere in which stress can be reduced and health enhanced.

Exercise

This is of course a key factor in reducing blood-pressure, as well as improving heart and circulatory health. It is vital that no one undertake vigorous exercise of any sort without first having a thorough check-up, and ideally an exercise tolerance test to assess how the heart and blood-pressure react to exercise. There is however one entirely safe form of exercise, and that is walking. Everyone who can walk should do so, and should do so regularly and methodically. Thus, it is safe to say that at least thirty minutes should be spent walking, at least every other day. The speed and distance involved should be dictated by the conditions, terrain, etc., that are available. Ideally walking should be on level ground, and the speed should be such as not to produce any distress at all. It should however result in a mild degree of heavy breathing. There should be no suggestion of any sensation of pain, constriction, or discomfort, in the chest, arms, neck, jaw, etc., during such walking. If there is, then medical attention is essential, as this *may* indicate that the heart muscles are inadequately supplied with blood. If however there is no such reaction, then a moderately brisk walk (not a jog, unless cleared by your medical adviser) at the intervals mentioned (more if possible) can only help. The long-term blood-pressure response to such increased activity is to reduce it, since the increased efficiency of the circulatory system, as a result of the muscular activity, reduces the load on the heart and helps the veins to reduce their back-pressure. If possible part of the walking exercise should be accompanied by the breathing exercise outlined later in this chapter.

Apart from walking, the use of a static bicycle, or

swimming, (in suitably warm water), are reasonable alternatives. Neither of these have the benefits of walking however, and they are only mentioned as safe, rather than as equally desirable. All competitive sport should be avoided for the duration of the anti-blood-pressure campaign.

Golf is sometimes suggested as a good way of getting some walking done. Its disadvantages include the tendency for a competitive edge to creep into it, as well as the fact that the walking involved is not continuous but is broken up into segments, with pauses to find, address and hit the ball. It is also frequently the case that golf courses are undulating, and a good deal of uphill walking is therefore called for. This may be undesirable. Walking is safe, extremely valuable, and essential as part of any programme for lowering blood-pressure when it is high, and keeping it normal.

Breathing Exercises

The use of controlled breathing is another vital element in the programme. As mentioned in earlier chapters, the circulation of blood round the body is assisted by the major pump mechanisms of the muscles and the diaphragm as it moves during the breathing cycle. The need to improve the mechanism of breathing is twofold: to assist in this dual pumping mechanism and to increase the amount of oxygen available, for the blood. This latter consideration is important inasmuch as the role of oxygen carrier played by the blood, can vitally affect the blood-pressure. If tissues are inadequately oxygenated, they send messages of distress, demanding more oxygen to be supplied. This leads to increased blood being pumped to meet the need, with all the consequences of strain on the heart, and increased pressure. If this is all being done against a background of tension on, or partial blockage of, the vessels carrying the blood so much the worse.

All in all, breathing exercises are an important part of the self-help measures involved in lowering the blood-pressure. The following exercises should be used so that two of them at least, are employed each day, as well as the one specifically designed to be used with walking.

Exercise One

Lie on your back with knees bent and shoulders and head supported by a cushion. Relax and breathe slowly but deeply in through the nose, allowing the air to fill the lower parts of the lungs. In doing so, the abdomen should be pushed downwards so that it gives the appearance of rising slightly above the lower level of the chest. It is essential that the air is allowed to flow to the bottom of the lungs. When the lower lung is filled with air, hold the position for a few seconds, and then slowly contract the abdomen and lower ribs, exhaling strongly at the same time. It is useful to count slowly to 4 or 5, as you breathe in, and after holding for one or two seconds, counting as you exhale, so that it takes slightly longer to breathe out than it took you to breathe in. Repeat ten to fifteen times.

Exercise Two

Stand upright. Take a deep breath through the nose, and bend slowly to the right, running your right hand down the outside of the leg and raising the left arm above your head, so that the body stretches to the right. As the movement is continued, more breath should be slowly drawn in. Now bend to the left, and allow the left hand to go down the left leg, and right arm to come over the head, to lever the body over to the left. During this movement, breathe out. Continue in this fashion, breathing in as you bend to the right and out as you bend to the left, ten times. The sequence of breathing should then be changed: breathe in as you bend to the left, and out when bending to the right. Do this ten times.

This exercise is designed to bring about increased expansion of the side of the chest. It is an excellent exercise to increase the drainage of the lungs, and to stimulate their eliminative action.

Exercise Three
Stand erect with your hands on the spine at the level of the waist; fingers should point towards the front of the body. Close your mouth and take in air, in small amounts, as if sniffing a flower. Continue to fill the lungs until no more can be taken. As you breathe in, bend the body gradually backward. When the chest is full expel the air slowly through the mouth, while at the same time bringing the body to the bending-forward position. This exercise requires practice. Do this ten to fifteen times.

Walking and Breathing Exercise
As well as performing at least two of the above daily (preferably all three, and ideally morning and evening) the following pattern can be adopted whilst walking. As you walk breathe in through the nose to a count of three, four or five steps, to fill the lungs. (The number will vary with the speed of walking, and your general

condition. Above all it must be a comfortable, unstrained, pattern.) Hold the breath for one or two strides and then exhale, still through the nose, to a count of two or three steps. *Note* that when doing breathing exercises, in a static situation (sitting, lying or standing) the breathing out phase should take slightly more time than breathing in; and when in an active phase (walking, swimming, etc.,) the reverse is true.

This pattern of counting and breathing as you walk, should only be carried out for a minute or two at a time, or until you find it difficult to maintain the rhythm. Repeat this several times during a half-hour walk.

As your fitness increases, and your lung capacity improves, so you will be able to do more and more of this type of controlled breathing during exercise. There is strong evidence of the value of the breathing exercise patterns described in reducing stress levels, and in helping to lower blood-pressure. The key to success lies in doing them as described, and in doing them regularly.

Relaxation Exercises
Relaxation exercises are most important in helping to bring stress down to acceptable levels. One, at least, of the following should be employed each day for not less than ten minutes, and if blood-pressure problems are evident, then twice daily is suggested. These should be done at a different time from the breathing exercises, when there is no likelihood of being disturbed. Find a quiet room and settle into a chair, or recline on a couch, or on the floor.

Breathing and Repeated Sound Technique
Sit or lie in a comfortable position in a suitable room.

Close your eyes and encourage a sense of heaviness and stillness. Focus your attention on the body, area by area, briefly, in order to assess them for obvious tension. Start with the feet and pass on to the lower legs, thighs, hips, buttocks, abdomen, lower back, chest, shoulders, neck, face, arms and hands. Do not overlook the eyes and jaw muscles. Many people screw up the eye muscles or clench the jaw habitually. If this is one of your traits, then pay particular attention to releasing these areas prior to continuing with the exercise.

This should only be a brief survey, not lasting for more than a few seconds in each region. As each area is visualized, any obvious tension should be released. If you are not sure whether a muscle or area is relaxed, tense it for a few seconds and then let it go. This brief but effective progressive muscular relaxation, area by area, prepares you for the exercise proper. It is worth emphasizing that relaxation is a passive act. You cannot 'try' to relax, for this is a contradiction in terms. Relaxation is a letting go, a switch off, which ideally involves no effort. Suggesting that dubious areas be tensed prior to 'letting go' is only to help to imprint on the mind the contrast between the two states. In this way, a gradual awareness will develop, enabling you to sense tension as it arises and, most importantly, to release it. (This is the basis of progressive muscular relaxation methods.)

For the purpose of this exercise the method outlined above is all that is required as preparation for the following breathing method.

Having spent a minute or, at most, two, in 'letting go' the obvious areas of tension in the musculature of the body, begin to breathe in and out through the nose.

Passively pay attention to your breathing and, as you breathe out, say silently and slowly to yourself any one-syllable word. Breathe in and out at any comfortable speed; there need be no rush, nor is there any need to make the breathing particularly slow. The rhythm should be as natural and unforced as possible, not particularly deep or unusually shallow.

You may well find that the rhythm will alter from time to time, or that periodically you will let out a very deep breath or sigh. Just let it happen, do not attempt to control the rhythm or depth of the respiration — simply use it to time the repetitive, slow enunciation of a word or sound. Many people use the word 'one' for this purpose, but any short word will do. Remember it should be said as you breathe out. This should continue for about ten minutes.

A feeling of stillness and calm should eventually be felt. In some cases a sense of happiness and deep relaxation is quickly achieved. In others there is only a gradual sense of being less stressed. In all cases where this type of exercise is performed as described, positive physiological changes will take place, irrespective of subjective feelings. In other words, there is a degree of stress reduction, whether or not you sense it from the outset.

Many people expect immediate, obvious changes. If disappointed in this expectation, they may abandon discipline involved in the regular performance of these exercises. This is sad and a waste, for it has been positively established that the benefits of the exercises often begin long before there is any awareness of improvement.

The repetition of the chosen word may well be

interrupted periodically by intrusive thoughts. When this happens, do not feel irritated, simply resume the use of the word to coincide with exhalation. Each individual will reap the benefits of this exercise at their own pace.

After about ten minutes of this exercise, stop repeating the word and simply allow the mind the luxury of doing nothing. Allow it to linger in the still, peaceful state to which you have drifted. Initially with the eyes closed and later with them open, spend at least two minutes in this state of inactivity. Slowly get up and resume your normal activities. (It is unwise to get up too quickly as over-oxygenation may result in transient giddiness.)

Progressive Muscular Relaxation

This method involves the systematic, conscious relaxation of all the body areas in sequence. The position for this exercise should be reclining — either on the floor or on a recliner-type chair. Ideally, there should be no distracting sounds and the clothing worn should not constrict in any way. (A few cycles of deep breathing should precede the exercise.)

Starting with the feet, try to sense or feel that the muscles of the area are not actively tense. Then deliberately tighten them, curling the toes under and holding the tension for five to ten seconds. Then tense the muscles even more strongly for a further few seconds before letting all the tension go and sensing the wonderful feeling of release. Try to register consciously what this feels like, especially in comparison with the tense state in which you have been holding them. Progress to the calf muscles and exercise them in the same way. First sense the state the muscles are in, then tense them, hold the position, and then tense them even more before letting go. Positively register the sense of release. In doing this to the leg muscles, there is a slight danger of inducing cramp. If this occurs stop testing that area immediately and move on to the next. After the calf muscles, go on to exercise the knees, then the upper leg, thigh muscles, the buttocks, the lower and upper back, the abdomen, the chest, the shoulders, the arms and hands, and then the neck, head and face. The precise sequence is irrelevant, as long as all these areas are 'treated' to the tensing, the extra tensing, and then the release.

Some areas need extra attention in this respect. The abdominal region is a good example. The tensing of these muscles can be achieved in either contraction (i.e. a pulling in of the muscles), or by stretching (i.e. a pushing outwards of the muscles). The variation in tensing method is applicable to many of the body's muscles. Indeed at different times, it is a good idea to vary the pattern, and instead of, for example, contracting and tensing a muscle group, try to stretch and tense them to their limit. This is especially useful in the muscles of the face, particularly in the mouth and eye region. Individual attention to these is important. On one occasion it would be desirable, for example, for the 'tensing' of the mouth muscles to take the form of holding the mouth open as widely as possible, with the lips tense during this phase. On a subsequent occasion, the 'tensing' could be a tight-pursed pressing together of the lips. If there is time available, both methods of tensing can be employed during the same exercise, especially in the areas you know to be very tense. The muscles controlling the jaw, eyes, mouth, tongue and neck are particularly important, as are the abdominal muscles, since much emotional tension is reflected in these regions, and release and relaxation often has profound effects.

There are between twenty and twenty-five of these 'areas', depending upon how you go about interpreting the guidelines given above; each should involve at least five to ten seconds of 'letting go' and of passively sensing that feeling. Thus, eight to ten minutes should suffice for the successful completion of this whole technique. This should be followed by several minutes of an unhurried return to a feeling of warm, relaxed tranquillity. Focus the mind on the whole body. Try to sense it as heavy and content, free of tension or effort. This might be enhanced by a few cycles of deep breathing. Stretch out like a cat, and then resume your normal activities.

Autogenic Exercises

True autogenic exercises need to be taught by a special teacher or practitioner well versed in this excellent system. The modified method outlined below is based on the work of the pioneer in this field Dr H. Schultz. The distinction between a relaxation exercise and a meditation technique is blurred at all times, but never more so than in autogenic methods, which are a blend of the two. At least fifteen and ideally twenty minutes should be given to the performance of this method. At another time of the day this, or another relaxation method, should also be performed again. This routine should become a welcome, eagerly anticipated oasis of calm and peace in the daily programme. Stress-proofing without such periods of 'switching off' is unlikely to be successfully achieved.

A reclining position should be adopted, with the eyes closed. External, distracting sounds should be minimized. The exercises involve the use of specific, verbalized messages to focus awareness on a particular area. No effort is involved, but simply a passive concentration on any sensations or emotions which may result from each message. Imagination or auto-suggestion has been found to have definite physiological effects. By combining a sequence of autogenic (i.e. self-generated) instructions, with the passive, focused aspect of meditation techniques, a powerful method of self-help has been created.

The exercise starts with a general thought, such as 'I am relaxed and at peace with myself'. Begin to breathe deeply in and out. Feel the light movement of the diaphragm and feel calm.

Stage I: The mind should focus on the area of the body to which the thought is directed. Start by silently verbalizing 'My right arm is heavy'. Think of the image of the right arm. Visualize it completely relaxed, and resting on its support (the floor, arm of the chair, etc.). Dissociate it from the body and from will-power. See the limp, detached arm as being heavy, having weight. After a few seconds the phrase should be repeated. This should be done a number of times before proceeding to the right leg, left leg, left arm, neck, shoulders and back. At each area, try to sense heaviness and maintain a passive feeling in the process.

Stage II: Again begin with the right arm, concentrating on it as you silently verbalize 'My right arm is warm'.

Repeat this and pause to sense warmth in the arm or hand. Repeat this several times. The pause should be unhurried. To encourage this feeling of warmth it may be useful to imagine that the sun's rays are shining onto the back of the hand warming it. The sensation of warmth spreads from there to the whole arm.

Proceed through all areas of the body, pausing for some seconds at each to assess sensations which may become apparent. Such changes as occur cannot be controlled, but will happen when the mind is in a passive, receptive state. This exercise increases the peripheral flow of blood, and relaxes the muscles controlling the blood-vessels. It is possible to increase measurably the temperature of an area of the body using these simple methods.

Stage III: The phrase 'I am alert and refreshed' ends the exercise. Breathe deeply, stretch, and continue the day's activities.

During stages I and II, the time spent in each area should not be less than about half a minute; it is however quite permissible to spend two or three minutes focusing on any one part, especially if the desired sensation of heaviness or warmth is achieved.

It will probably be found that the desired sensation is more easily sensed in one stage than another, and that some areas seem more 'responsive' than others. This is normal. It is also quite normal for there to be no subjective appreciation of any of the verbalized sensations. Do not worry about this. Even if nothing at all is sensed for some considerable time, possibly months, there is a great deal actually taking place within the body as a result of the whole exercise. Persistence, patience and a total lack of urgency is all that is necessary for this method to lead to a decrease in muscular tension and a sense of calm and well-being. A side-effect of this particular method is frequently experienced in terms of much improved peripheral circulation, i.e. an end to cold hands and feet.

Biofeedback

Biofeedback is a system which utilizes the 'feedback' to the individual of biological information not usually available to him, thus enabling him to learn to exercise control over organs and functions which are normally outside his voluntary control. By means of these techniques, individuals have achieved control over circulatory functions, as evidenced by the ability to increase the temperature of a particular body area. Other examples include control of the heart rate, blood-pressure, gastric secretions, brainwave patterns, skin resistance to electricity, relaxation of muscle groups, and so on. The effects of this system are profound, since such control has previously only been achieved using drug therapy.

The simplest biofeedback equipment is that which measures the electrical skin resistance (E.S.R.). Electrode pads are attached to the palm or fingers of either hand. The information derived via the electrodes is fed into a machine; this, in turn, produces a sound which is louder when the E.S.R. is low (indicating anxiety or tension), and softer when it is high (indicating calm and relaxation). The objective is to use the mind to silence the machine. This is achieved by trial and error until the individual learns what to do to reduce the sound level completely. At this point a relative state of relaxation will have been achieved. The control of blood-pressure and heart rate can be achieved in a similar way.

What is not certain is whether, in the long-term, the individual, having 'learned' to achieve the desired result whilst attached to biofeedback equipment, can continue to do so in everyday life. Other systems, such as meditation and relaxation techniques, do have the ability to influence every day experience, as well as allowing the possibility of increased 'awareness' and personality development. Biofeedback cannot, as yet, make similar claims. The best results with biofeedback have been achieved when such methods are combined with meditation and relaxation exercises.

Simple biofeedback equipment to monitor E.S.R. or skin temperature is available for around £50.00. No explicit instructions as to what to do to achieve the desired result, whether it be raising or lowering the temperature, or raising the E.S.R., are provided. The essence of the technique is for the individual to learn, by repetition, what it is that has to be done, using the mind to silence the buzzer or to switch off the light on the machine. It is a system which requires internal experimentation and, initially, the results might well be chaotic, as noises get louder in response to 'wrong' signals. From infancy onwards, we all learn to function in a very similar manner.

Nutrition
Nutrition is the major key to reducing high blood-pressure, and it is this area which calls for your most dedicated efforts. You will find set out the key factors in the diet which are undesirable as far as building up

problems which can result in hypertension. These include refined products (white flour, sugar, etc.), fats, which contribute to free radical activity and consequent damage to blood-vessel walls, as well as resulting (with refined foods) in overweight situations, which are a major factor in hypertension development. Fats of course also add to the substances which become part of the clogging process in the arteries. Eating excessive quantities of meat has been shown to be a key factor, as has the use of sodium-rich foods, especially salt (in certain people). The use of alcohol too must be modified. This leaves a diet in which the foods that need to be emphasized as being helpful include the low-fat proteins, such as fish, poultry (not the skin though), and low-fat cheese; all vegetables and fruits, and the whole range of grains, seeds, nuts (unsalted and not roasted) as well as all the pulse family, with the wonderful flavours and textures that this offers.

The dietary pattern that is outlined below should be adopted over a period of several weeks, rather than overnight. The closer you can get to it the better. Not all foods are suitable for all people, and tastes differ greatly. Within the general outline and choices described, there is ample opportunity for finding an individual pattern. At the end of this section you will find notes on fasting. The use of simple short fasts (24-36 hours), as well as the occasional 2 or 3 day fast, helps enormously in preparing the body for the detoxification and regeneration which is so vital to renewed health and vigour. The following are a list of general dietary guidelines followed by a list of foods to avoid (with suggested alternatives), and then an outline of a menu which can be adapted to your own needs and tastes.

General Rules of Eating and Diet

1. Digestion begins in the mouth. Food should be eaten slowly and chewed thoroughly.
2. Avoiding foods that are very hot or very cold will improve digestive functions.
3. Drinking any liquid with meals interferes with digestion, as does any liquid taken up to an hour after a main meal.
4. Simple meals, without sauces, are easier to digest. Combinations of certain foods can produce indigestion, e.g. protein and carbohydrate do not mix well (bread and cheese or fish and chips).
5. Fried and roasted foods are difficult to digest and should play little or no part in the diet.
6. Foods to avoid:
   * All white flour products, such as white bread, cakes, pasta, pastry, biscuits. Replace with wholemeal alternatives.
   * All sugar of any kind, and its products, such as sweets, jams, soft drinks, ices, etc. Replace with fruit, dried fruit, sugarless jam, fresh fruit juice, fruit flavoured natural yogurt, etc.
   * Polished (white) rice. Replace with unpolished (brown) rice.
   * Any foods containing additives, preservatives, colouring, etc., such as most tinned foods.
   * Tea, coffee, chocolate. Replace with herb teas, dandelion or other coffee substitutes.
   * Strong condiments (vinegar, pickles, pepper, curry, etc.). Replace with herbs.
   * Milk, butter, cream and their derivatives. Use only low-fat cheese in moderation. Natural yogurt or sour milk (acidophilus milk).

* Margarine.
* Salt and salted foods.
* Meat. If animal protein is to be eaten then fish and chicken (no skin) etc. are more desirable than red meat. Eat no more than four eggs weekly.
7. Foods to include:
    * Drinks: Herb teas (red clover, spring water, sage, camomile, etc.). Coffee substitute (pioneer, caro, dandelion). Fresh unsweetened fruit juice and vegetable juices. Nut/soya milk.
    * Cereals: Millet, oatmeal, unpolished rice, buckwheat, barley, rye or wholemeal bread, sprouted grains (wheat).
    * Proteins: Fish, chicken, liver, occasional lean meat.
    * Beans: Chickpeas, lima, soya, lentils, etc.
    * Sweeteners: A little honey, date sugar or maple syrup.
    * Fruits: Apples, bananas, pears, avocados, cherries, apricots, peaches, nectarines, pawpaw. If possible organically grown and unsprayed. Dried fruit (if sun-dried).
    * Nuts: Walnuts, almonds, pecans, hazels, unsalted peanuts.
    * Vegetables: All vegetables. Freshly frozen vegetables.
    * Seasoning: Parsley, chives, garlic, sage, marjoram, thyme, oregano, powdered kelp, vegetable seasoning (without salt). Salt substitute such as potassium chloride.
    * Seeds: Sunflower, pumpkin, sesame, apple, nectarine, pear.
    * Sprouting seeds and beans: Mung beans, wheat sprouts, alfalfa, etc. Include these in salads or use as

a sandwich filler.
* Soups: Include any vegetables, plus beans, millet, cereals, (no meat or fat stock).
8. Forbidden Foods:
Tap water.
Tea, coffee, alcohol, bottled soft drinks.
Processed cereals, i.e. flaked, puffed, etc. All white flour products.
Fat meat, bacon, pork, ham, tinned or smoked meat, salted meat.
Cane or beet sugar, artificial sweeteners.
Butter, full-fat milk, cream, full fat cheese.
Tinned fruit, sulphur dried fruit.
Roasted or salted nuts or peanuts.
Tinned vegetables.
Salt, pepper, curry, chillies, etc.
Salted or roasted seeds.
Tinned, packet or block soups.

General Menu Sheet
Breakfast: Choose from:
1. Oatmeal porridge (without salt or sugar) and honey if desired.
2. Muesli (oats, nuts and dried fruit mixture) moistened with fruit juice or natural yogurt. Add a little honey if desired.
3. Wholemeal bread or toast. Butter with honey or yeast spread.
4. Fresh fruit and/or soaked or lightly cooked dried fruit (no sugar).

Drink herb tea or coffee substitute or fresh fruit juice. Try never to miss eating at least one of the above, and ideally two. Breakfast is a very important meal in balancing the body's metabolism.

On three days a week you may eat a boiled or poached egg for breakfast as well.

Midmorning:
Fresh fruit or unsalted nuts or herb tea.

Lunch:
Ideally this meal should mainly be a salad meal. If it is not, then the evening meal should contain a large mixed salad. Use as many ingredients as are in season. Dress with lemon juice and olive oil (no vinegar or salt). Add wholemeal bread or a brown rice savoury, or a baked potato (in its skin). A small amount of low-fat cheese may be added, but it should be remembered that this meal is meant mainly to be a salad and carbohydrate meal.

Evening meal:
This meal should mainly be protein such as fish or chicken (not the skin) or liver or, no more than once a week, red meat (lean) or a vegetarian combination of pulses (beans) and cereals (such as brown rice). Add to this fresh vegetables or salad.

Dessert:
Fresh fruit.

This pattern of eating should be followed for not less than six months in order to achieve a degree of control of blood-pressure. Do not expect results inside the first two months though it is thus advisable not to keep checking the pressure. Results will come but the reversal of a major trend towards ill health does take time, and you must give the body a chance. When a reasonable level of blood-pressure is achieved, the knowledge gained by this whole exercise in self-help will enable you to maintain it, by adapting the diet and relaxing only slightly the pattern described above.

Supplements

These are known to be helpful in reducing blood-pressure, and aid cardiovascular function. Include the following:

Vitamin C with Bioflavonoids — 1g daily.

Vitamin E (d-Alpha tocopherol) — 200 to 400 iu daily.

Vitamin B complex (a formula which contains at least 25mg each of vitamins B_1, B_2, nicotinamide (B_3), calcium pantothenate (B_5) and Pyridoxine (B_6) — 1 daily.

As an alternative to this 8 brewer's yeast tablets can be taken daily.

Magnesium — 500mg daily.*

Potassium — 150mg daily.*

Manganese — 50mg daily.*

Selenium — 50mg daily.

Garlic capsules — 2 daily.

Bromelaine enzymes (pineapple derivative) — one 200mg tablet twice daily before food.

---

* These should be obtained in the orotate form (which is described on the container as B_{13} magnesium, for example) as this ensures easy assimilation.

Glutathione (amino acid compound)* — 500mg twice daily.

Chelation

Deposits of calcium in the arteries can be removed by the oral route as well as the more efficient, but more difficult, intravenous method discussed on page 49. The following is an outline of the pattern of supplement- ation recommended by Dr Morton Walker and Dr Garry Gordon, in their book *The Chelation Answer* (Evans, 1982). They suggest a variety of nutrients which interact to chelate cholesterol and calcium deposits out of the arterial walls. Taking such high levels of supplements should be achieved over a period of several months, and should not be started immediately. Begin with about a quarter of the dosages recommended, and slowly build up to the required level, maintaining this for six months or so. The dietary pattern, outlined previously, should be maintained throughout this programme, together with exercise and other recom- mendations. These supplements should replace those suggested above, not be in addition to them.

Chelation Programme:
4g Lecithin.
1 tablespoon Wheatgerm (source of vitamin E).
500mg oil of Evening Primrose (or 12g sunflower

---

* This is to assist in the removal of free radicals from the system. It, and the other supplements, are totally non-toxic at these dosages. The B_{13} minerals (magnesium, potassium, etc.) as well as the bromelaine enzymes, and glutathione can be obtained from Larkhall Laboratories, 225 Putney Bridge Road, London SW15, or from a health food store.

seeds) as a source of linoleic acid.

4g of vitamin C.

50mg of niacin (vitamin B_3), three times daily.

250mg vitamin B_{15} (also known as Dimethylglycine, DMG).

1 strong vitamin B-complex tablet.

100mg selenium.

1g magnesium (as magnesium orotate, or B_{13} magnesium).

20mg manganese (as manganese orotate or B_{13} manganese).

600mg bromelaine.

6 to 10 garlic capsules.

High fibre foods such as pulses, whole grains and all vegetables and fruits, are an essential part of the chelation from the body of excess cholesterol.

Following such a programme of chelation as that outlined above calls for a certain dedication, and it is not inexpensive. It is possible to modify the programme and that is what I have suggested in the list of supplements which preceded the discussion of the chelation programme.

One other major method exists by which the self-healing characteristics of the body can be encouraged, and that is fasting, which we will consider next.

6.

Fasting for Health

Fasting is the oldest method of healing. It is instinctive in sick animals, and probably was in primitive man too. If carried out sensibly, fasting can also be useful in preventing disease.

Fasting is often confused with starvation, but strictly speaking it is abstinence for a given time from solid food, but not from liquids. It is the use of liquids that is the controversial area. Some experts say fasting is effective only if it is undertaken on water only, whereas others, including myself, would advocate that fasting should be undertaken using fruit and vegetable juices. Opinion also differs on how long a fast should continue; this largely depends on whether it is being employed to treat ill health, as a method of preventive medicine, or simply to improve health. For most people a few days of fasting can do nothing but good and can often mean the beginning of recovery from ill health. It is imperative, however, that no one attempts a long fast unless they are under the supervision of the experienced practitioner.

Fasting is useful in most cases of physical illness, but there are certain circumstances where it should not be used. Anyone —

with an ulcer,

with a history of gout,

who is pregnant,

who is diabetic,

who has heart disease,

who has kidney disease,

who has cancer,

should seek professional advice before trying any self-treatment with fasting.

This warning does not mean that fasting is unsuitable for these conditions, but it does mean that expert help is required to decide on the type of fast, and how long it should be maintained.

There are some strange things that might happen to the body during a fast, and it is best to understand them before beginning so that there is no anxiety when these things happen; they are after all, signs of rejuvenation.

The sort of signs you can expect to notice are: furred tongue, bad breath, dark and often offensive urine, and sometimes the voiding of amazing accretions from the bowels. The degree and intensity of the signs of the body cleansing itself of accumulated toxic waste will vary greatly from person to person, often depending on the underlying health and vitality of the individual, as well as the type of fast being used. Surprisingly, hunger is often not noticed after the first day.

Fasting can be seen as a preparation for spontaneous self-healing by the body. It is not a cure for anything but it is providing the body with a chance to eliminate toxins which are preventing the body from healing itself. So it is important not to treat the initial signs of fasting, such as a 'sick' headache, with any drugs or potions that will suppress them. The headache will go and the tongue will again become pink and healthy. All other symptoms will disappear too. A short fast may not be long enough for all these things to happen but by repetition the intensity of elimination of the first fast will disappear until, in time, fasts may be enjoyed without marked symptoms, which is a sign of increased health.

An area of controversy in fasting is the use of enemas, colonic irrigation and laxatives. There are times when one of these may be called for. If however there is no history of constipation, and general health is good, then enemas, etc. are not necessary. But if a chronic illness is involved, especially of the bowel, or an allergic or catarrhal condition, then there is a good case for daily enemas or a herbal laxative before and after the short fast. There are no hard and fast rules, but it is important to recognize that the state of health of the bowel largely determines the degree of health of the body. Health is impossible without a healthy digestive system, and fasting is one of the best ways of encouraging this. Supplements of 'friendly' bacteria to the bowel are a further aid to healthy digestion. Breaking the fast correctly is also important. After any length of time without solid food there must be a gentle transition back to full diet.

It is also important that during a fast some exercise is taken; staying in bed is seldom called for, but plenty of rest is necessary. So it is unwise to fast while carrying on normal work. It is also unwise to drive during a fast because dizziness may occur. Fresh air and rest are important, as is the avoidance of stress, which explains the popularity of health farms and hydros, which can offer a restful environment.

Three day fasts, done over a weekend, are a good introduction, and there is one set out below. But it is necessary to set aside a weekend for the fasting, during which you drop all major obligations and duties. A three day detoxification every four to six weeks, over six or twelve months will provide a dramatic improvement in health in most people, and will help normalize hypertension.

Alternatively you might prefer to fast for one day each week. A light meal can be eaten midday on a Saturday, followed by juice on Saturday evening through to Sunday evening, with the fast being broken Sunday evening or Monday morning. This 24 to 36-hour fast every week or fortnight will also be beneficial to health.

In all cases the aim of a fast is to rest the body from the constant onslaught of food, so the principles of a fast can also be applied to everyday eating to make us feel more vital and lively. For instance, breakfast implies that we have been, for a period, without food. This is true if the last meal of the day was at 6pm and breakfast is at 7 or 8am. But if we eat after 9 at night then the digestive system will barely have finished coping with the evening meal before the next food starts to arrive. Such a pattern of eating makes people sluggish and lethargic. By eating earlier in the evening, with no snacks later on, you can be livelier in the morning and have a rested digestive system ready for the next day. Remember, longer fasts should only be undertaken with the help of a qualified nutritionally-orientated health practitioner.

Preparing for a fast:

The day before: a herbal laxative such as psyllium seeds, or a broth made of flax seed (linseed), or castor oil should be taken after the midday meal, which should itself be light (vegetarian for preference, such as a mixed salad or a vegetable soup).

In the evening: have a light fruit meal (pears, apple, grapes, or a vegetable broth (see recipe below).

Vegetable Broth Recipe

Use organically grown vegetables if possible. If not, scrub well before use. Into 4 pints (2.2 litres/10 cups) of spring water place four cupfuls finely chopped beetroots, carrots, thick potato peelings, parsley, courgette, and leaves of beetroot or parsnip. Use no sulphur-rich vegetables which might produce gas, such as cabbage or onions. Simmer for five minutes over a low heat to allow for the breakdown of the vegetable fibre and the release of nutrients into the liquid. Cool and strain, using only the liquid and not the left over vegetable content. Don't add salt, as this broth will contain ample natural minerals which are rapidly absorbed thus providing nutrients without straining the digestive system. Also, it is alkaline and neutralizes any acidity resulting from the fast. Drink at least one pint (570ml/2½ cups) of this broth daily during the fast.

On rising the next day: drink either camomile or peppermint tea (unsweetened); or a cup of vegetable broth, or a cup of half spring water and carrot juice, beetroot juice, or warm or cold apple juice.

A selection of one of these items or bottled spring water, should be consumed at two- to three-hourly intervals during the day, making sure that vegetable broth is consumed at least twice during the day (not less than one pint daily) and that the total liquid intake is not less than two and a half pints, and not more than four pints daily.

If fresh vegetable juice is not obtainable, then *Biotta* vegetable juice is available at most health food stores, and is suitable for use in fasting as it contains no preservatives (other than lactic acid) and is guaranteed organically grown. Carrot and beetroot are the ideal juices. Continue this pattern for the two or three days of the fast.

Finish the fast by eating, on the evening of the final day, one of the following 'meals': Puréed cooked apple or pear; puréed carrot plus a little puréed vegetable soup; live natural yogurt can be eaten with either of these choices. Chew all food very thoroughly and slowly.

The next morning eat yogurt and grated apple, or a fresh pear meal, and have a salad and jacket potato for the lunch meal, continuing thereafter on a normal pattern of eating.

The advice for ending a fast depends upon a person not being sensitive to any of the foods mentioned. If dairy produce, for example, is in any way suspect then it should play no part in breaking a fast. For this reason, anyone with suspected allergies should take advice, or be under some degree of supervision during this time.

If it is possible, a herbal laxative or castor oil should be used on the last evening of the fast, or a warm water enema should be used. If the individual involved is chronically ill, then daily, small warm water enemas should be used during the fast. The hygiene of the bowel can be further improved by employing one or all of the following during the fast, and for a week or so afterwards:

Daily take a quarter teaspoon of *Vital-Dophilus** or half a teaspoon of *Super-Dophilus.***

These highly concentrated acidophilus products will enhance the flora of the bowel while the *Vital-Dophilus* is suitable for people who are milk sensitive.

Stir a teaspoon of fine green clay powder*** into a small glass of spring water and allow it to settle, for an hour. Drink the water, but not the sediment. Do this at least once a day during the fast, and for a week after. The clay has a detoxifying quality and soothes the bowel.

Expect to feel lethargic during the fast, and perhaps a little colder than usual, so wear an extra layer of clothing! Rest as much as possible, since the whole object is to allow energy to be employed towards healing, not diffused in unnecessary activity. Take no medication of any sort.

In people of normal weight the fast will result in a number of predictable and beneficial effects, but it won't have the same physiological response in very overweight individuals. For example, growth hormone

* *Vital-Dophilus* from Klaire laboratories, 126 Acomb Road, York YO1 4EY.
** *Super-Dophilus* from G & G Supplies, 175 London Road, East Grinstead, Sussex RH19 1YY.
*** Fine green clay is available from Cantassium Co., 225-229 Putney Bridge Road, London SW15.

is released by the pituitary as a response to fasting in individuals of normal weight, but less so in the overweight (growth hormone has many functions, including fat mobilization). Thus, if the fast is undertaken for weight control, it must of necessity be a long fast, and it is vital that this is under strict supervision. A short fast, by an overweight person is quite in order, provided their general health is stable.

Fasting is safe if employed correctly and is one of the swiftest detoxifying and health promoting methods available. Try it regularly, and you will probably be hooked on it for life, which, if animal studies are any guide, will be longer than if you do not fast regularly.

Blood-pressure is certain to drop during a fast, and with repetition as outlined — together with the other measures already discussed — you now have a self-help programme which can give you extra years of healthy life with a stable blood-pressure.

INDEX